The 30 Day Difference
CLEAN EATING PLAN

"A Strategic Meal Plan Guide for Rapid Weight Loss"

by Marlee Gray

Send testimonials to:

Marlee Gray

P.O.Box 893
Woodstock GA. 30188

www.30daydifferencechallenge.com

CONTENTS

This publication contains the opinions and ideas of its author. This book is intended as a reference manual to provide helpful information. This is not a medical guide or substitute for medical advice. It is sold with the understanding that the author and publisher are not rendering medical, health, or any other kind of professional services in the book. The reader should consult with his or her doctor or medical professional before adopting any of the suggestions or methods in this book.

The author and publisher specifically disclaim all responsibility for any liability, loss or risk, personal or otherwise, which is incurred as a consequence, directly or indirectly as the results of the use or applications of any of the contents in this book.

Mention of specific brand name products, companies, organizations, people, quotes or authorities in this book does not imply endorsement by the author or publisher, nor does mention of specific brand name products, companies, organizations, people or authorities imply that they endorse this book, its author or the publisher. The brand name products mentioned in this book are trademarks or registered trademarks of the respective companies.

Library of Congress Cataloging-in-Publication Data is Available Upon Request

This book is dedicated to anyone who has suffered from or overcome illness, depression, loss or obesity. You are needed, you are strong and you are loved.

INTRODUCTION

Welcome to The 30 Day Difference Challenge: A healthy eating program plan that will challenge you to improve your habits and change your life. If you've ever been sick, bloated, extremely tired, restless, stressed, overweight, fought disease, suffered from hormonal imbalance or mental blocks, this program is for you!

Before I became a nutrition coach, I suffered from all of the above. Growing up, I ate a lot of food associated with special occasions, holidays and celebrations. Like most, I looked forward to "treating" myself, but eating bad foods was no way to treat or reward myself at all. After developing IBS, and a plethora of health issues that I could no longer manage, I decided to take my health into my own hands. After years of extensive research and testing, The 30 Day Difference Clean Eating Plan was developed. The very last time I went to the doctor before doing this meal plan, my swelling, weight gain and hormones were out of control. I knew I needed help that went beyond medication but lacked the motivation and structure to do something. I had been working out for months and years off and on but lacked seeing true results. It was frustrating, overwhelming, discouraging and for a moment I accepted that maybe being sick and overweight was my fate but I wanted to try at least one more time.

Once The 30 Day Difference menu plan was developed, it was convenient to follow. I immediately noticed reduced swelling, drastic fat loss, clarity in my mind and acne vanishing. I was even healed from a long-term illness! The moment I was able to fit into jeans I hadn't worn since before giving birth years prior, I knew that this plan truly made a difference. My energy was through the roof and I wanted to share the experience with others. The results from the test group were mind blowing with some people literally losing 10-11 pounds the first week with no exercise. Not just water weight, but fat loss. We have had countless non-scale victories as well, which makes this program so unique. Although doing this plan will subsequently cause healthy weight loss, the benefits of this specific combination of nutrition will truly make a difference in other areas of your health.

So here's the thing, for years, we've been told that certain foods are good for us and provide the nutrients we need but the truth of the matter is sometimes even foods that are deemed healthy are not good for your particular body. The 30 Day Difference Clean Eating Plan was designed to help you gain proper knowledge in nutrition, healthy meal prep and transform your way of thinking from a temporary diet to a healthy lifestyle. As you go on this journey over the next 30 days, my hope is that you are inspired, empowered, improve your health, achieve your goals and even above weight loss, truly see a difference in your life. Happy 30 Day!

CHAPTER ONE
What is the 30 Day Difference Plan?

Well let's start with what it's not. The 30DD Plan is not a diet. So get it out of your head right now that you are sacrificing flavorful food to trade in for cardboard. And even if it was a diet, it's just 30 days. So what's sacrificing crappy meals for a healthy deal? The trade off is simple, you get to experience the best health of your life and rid yourself of harmful toxins, cravings and unnecessary ailments caused by unhealthy eating. So instead of deciding to try this program, get excited about doing this program. It's time to go from trying to doing and this plan will help you with a mindset transformation and your relationship with food.

"We overeat and eat the wrong things to fulfill an emotional trigger in our minds yet we eat right and get healthy to fulfill the needs of our bodies. This is often a constant battle but ultimately being consistent in fulfilling the proper needs for our bodies will help condition the shape of our minds. If you finally go from having a desire to making a decision to get healthy, in the end, you win. " –K.M.

Now that you're all in, and ready to win, let's talk about what this program really is and how it benefits you.

About The 30 DD Plan:

The 30 Day Difference Plan is a meal plan program focused on a strategic combination of healthy low glycemic index foods aiding in self discipline, disease prevention and portion control. The meal plan is to be followed closely plugging in foods from the provided food list every day of the week. One of the best parts of this program is that you get to create your own healthy meals based on the meal plan rubric. This encourages you to explore food and nutrition like never before, discovering more flavors, herbs and taste without the overwhelming amounts of chemicals, additives, pollutants, sugar, salts and unhealthy fats that can be detrimental to your health. When you have cravings, your body is typically deficient in a specific vitamin or mineral. Your palette will adjust quickly and you will begin to crave good unprocessed foods that your body needs on a daily basis to function at its best. This program is affordable, easy to follow and almost anyone can do it. That anyone means you!

How Does it Work?

It's simple. In this book you will find your approved food list. Take the list to the grocery store and buy the food items on it. If it's not on the list, don't buy it. There will be days where you can begin adding in additional condiments and herbs, but most of these items are already stocked in your cabinets or refrigerator. Each day you can look forward to eating three healthy meals and snacks along with a special drink to help flush fat and toxins. Exercise is not mandatory on this program but aids in healthy blood flow and increased fat loss while participating.

What are the Benefits?

Anytime that you fuel your body with nutrients, something amazing begins to happen, especially with the food combination from The 30 Day Difference Plan. The benefits of this plan includes but are not limited to:

Weight Loss

Regulated Blood Sugar

Balance of Hormones

Mental Clarity

Appetite Control

Detox of Toxins and Free Radicals

Disease Prevention

Boost in Energy/ Endurance

Boost in Metabolism

Decreased Bloating

Lowered Blood Pressure

Improved Immune System

Reduced Stress/Anxiety

Lower Cholesterol

Better Sleep

Improved Lung Function and Breathing

Reduced Allergies

Anti Aging

Better Reproductive System

Improved Libido

CHAPTER TWO
Why Should I Participate?

Didn't we just mention weight loss? So if that isn't enough, here's more. If you have ever dealt with any of the problems mentioned in the introduction of this book then this is the perfect plan for you. You will see fast results and start feeling better immediately. If you're on the go but don't have time to eat right, this is also the plan for you. We've had participates from law enforcement, stay at home moms, nurses, teachers, salesmen, music professionals, human resources professionals, retirees, CEO's, entrepreneurs and more complete this plan with major success. All you have to do is plug in the foods from the provided menu and the weight loss is inevitable.

The World Health Organization stated an unhealthy diet is one of the major risk factors for a range of chronic diseases, including cardiovascular diseases, cancer, diabetes and other conditions linked to obesity. Statistics show that 65 percent of people gain weight back within three years of dieting according to Dr. Foster at University of Pennsylvania. Thankfully, this is not a diet but a healthy eating meal plan that can be implemented as a lifestyle. With this plan and support from other participates you are guaranteed to succeed. As a matter of fact, most people fail at reaching health goals due to lack of accountability or support. You know the old saying, "Teamwork makes the dream work?" Well, getting friends, co-workers and family members to join you on this plan is a great way to keep you accountable as well. We would love to have them a part of The 30 Day Difference Family!

The amazing thing about The 30 Day Difference Plan is that it comes with a great deal of support and additional health perks by joining the online community from the Facebook Group. There you will find additional meal ideas, frequently asked questions, guidance tools, videos and more. For additional support and guidance we encourage you to join our Facebook group at:

www.facebook.com/groups/30DayDifferenceChallenge

#30DDPLAN

CHAPTER THREE
Getting Started

In the words of Vince Lombardi, "Most people fail, not because of lack of desire, but, because of lack of commitment." The main thing you need to start and successfully complete this program is strong commitment to follow through. If you stumble, it doesn't mean you failed, so pick up on the next meal and keep going. On this plan it's okay if you have an, "oh crap" moment, just don't let it turn into a, "screw it" moment where you mess up once and decide to keep doing damage. Just because you make a mistake, doesn't mean your eating plan has to be ruined.

The first three days of the meal plan are identical to help detox your body and jumpstart your clean eating. Your body may experience slight changes, which is normal due to toxins being released and flushed out of your system. Don't let that deter you and please don't fret, within a couple of days you will feel a burst of energy and the hardest part will be out of the way. The first day of recommended exercise is day four. As far as grocery shopping, not everything on the list needs to be purchased all at once. For the best shopping strategy, skim ahead in the book to look at the menu week by week. If ever in doubt about what to eat, remember the general rule of thumb is, if it's not on the food list, you can't have it. Please see below for some key tips to help you get started and succeed on The 30 DD Plan:

TIPS

✓ Season food with only no salt herbs and/or provided salt option.

✓ Weigh in once a week at the beginning of the week first thing in the morning.

✓ Preferred Day for Weigh In is Monday.

✓ No skipping food or meals on the plan.

✓ Eggs and citric fruit can be substituted for HEALTH reasons only. See Facebook group for details.

✓ If hunger occurs in between meals, you may always add additional vegetables.

✓ Drink plenty of purified water.

✓ Take a before and after photo.

✓ Take measurements on your first and last day.

✓ Set small goals for yourself and track progress.

So that is how you participate in The 30 Day Difference Clean Eating Plan aka #30DDPlan in a nutshell. You can now turn the page to get started on one of best health journeys of your life. The time has finally come for change. You've got a made up mind and this time you will succeed and see a difference. Grab the grocery list on the next page and head to the store. See you at the end of your 30 days!

LET'S GET STARTED!

Grocery Food Check List

- ☐ Coconut Oil
- ☐ Olive Oil
- ☐ Pink Himalayan or Sea Salt
- ☐ Organic Apple Cider Vinegar "With Mother"
- ☐ Lemons
- ☐ Cucumber
- ☐ Fresh Mint Leaves
- ☐ Fresh Basil Leaves
- ☐ Ginger root
- ☐ Turmeric (Powder)
- ☐ Mrs. Dash No Salt Seasoning
- ☐ Eggs or Egg White Substitute
- ☐ Frozen Berries
- ☐ Frozen Pineapple
- ☐ Oranges
- ☐ Grapefruit
- ☐ Green Apples
- ☐ Avocado
- ☐ Spinach and Leafy Greens (No Iceberg)
- ☐ Green Vegetables (No Asparagus, Green Beans, Peas or Cabbage)
- ☐ Romaine Lettuce Boats for Wraps
- ☐ Sweet Potatoes
- ☐ Almond, Coconut or Cashew Milk (No Dairy or Soy)
- ☐ Oatmeal
- ☐ Brown Rice, Quinoa or Amaranth
- ☐ Raw/Unsalted Cashews or Almonds
- ☐ Dried Dates or Prunes
- ☐ Larabars (No Chocolate or Peanut Butter)
- ☐ Almond Butter-No Sugar Added
- ☐ Lean Poultry (No Beef , Pork, Crabmeat, Shrimp or Shellfish)
- ☐ Skinless Chicken
- ☐ Skinless Turkey Breast
- ☐ Ground Turkey
- ☐ Skinless Fish
- ☐ Salad Dressing (Oil Based, No Fructose Corn Syrup)
- ☐ Dark Chocolate
- ☐ Chia Seeds
- ☐ Green Tea
- ☐ Purified Water
- ☐ Alkaline Water *Optional

FOODS & DRINKS TO AVOID

The general rule of thumb is, if it's not on the approved food list, don't eat it. There are, however, a few exceptions to this rule. If you refer back to Chapter 2, we discuss cooking your foods with herbs that have no salt contents. Onions and garlic are acceptable garnishes as well. Over the next 30 days please avoid these foods and drinks:

Butter

Sugar

Honey

Coffee

Soda/Juice

Shellfish

Processed Foods

Fried Foods

Canned Meat and Canned Vegetables

Dairy (Eggs Allowed)

Bread

Corn

Beans

Legumes

Peanut Butter

Pasta

Wheat/Gluten

Alcohol

Junk Food

Bell Peppers

Mushrooms

Hot Sauce/Spicy Seasonings

Beef

Pork

Soy

FAT FLUSH DRINK

This combination in a cup of purified water helps to flush out toxins that get released as your body gets a reset. If you have sensitivity to acid go with Option Two. This drink can be sipped off of the whole morning up until lunchtime. Do not sip past lunchtime to avoid oral sensitivity or any imbalances. Avoid using alkaline water with Option One.

OPTION #1

(1) Small Lemon (Sliced)

(2-3) Mint Leaves

(1) Basil Leaf

(1/3) Cucumber (Sliced)

(1-2) Caps Organic Apple Cider Vinegar

(16oz) Purified Water

OPTION #2

(1/3) Cucumber (Sliced)

(2-3) Mint Leaves

(1-2) Basil Leaves

(1) Ginger Root

(16oz) Purified Water or

(16oz) Alkaline Water

BERRY or TANGY APPLE KIWI SMOOTHIE

The smoothie option steps into play on day four, the same day that it's safe to introduce light exercise into the program. Although you may still be a little full from breakfast, this smoothie is great to sip off of for satiety and energy/strength. You will start off with only the Berry Smoothie for Week One. During the weeks to come, you can rotate which smoothie you drink weekly for different benefits.

Berry Smoothie Recipe
(Option for Weeks 1-4)

(8oz) Substitute Milk or Purified Water
(1 Cup) Frozen Mixed Berries
(1 Cup) Frozen Pineapple
(1 Cup) Spinach
(2 TBSP) Chia Seeds

Tangy Apple Kiwi Smoothie Recipe
(Option for Weeks 2-4)

(8oz) Purified Water
(1) Small/Medium Sliced Green Apple
(1/2) Celery Stalk
(1) Kiwi
(1 Cup) Kale or Spinach
(2-3) Cilantro Stems
(2 TBSP) Chia Seeds
(1/3 Cup) Frozen Pineapple

SAMPLE MENU
DAY 1

Breakfast	Fat Flush Drink 3 Boiled Egg Whites 1/2 Grapefruit
Lunch	5 oz Baked Flounder 2 Cups Sautéed Kale w/ Garlic
Snack	Larabar
Dinner	4 oz Pan Seared Grouper 1 Cup Spinach w/ Oil Dressing 1 Cup Grilled Zucchini

SAMPLE MENU
DAY 4

Breakfast	Fat Flush Drink 3 Boiled Egg Whites 1/2 Cup Oatmeal 1/4 Cup Berries
Snack	Berry Smoothie
Lunch	4 oz Ground Turkey Burger 1 Cup of Kale w/ Onions and Dressing ½ Baked Sweet Potato
Snack	½ Orange
Dinner	4 oz Ground Turkey 2 Lettuce Wraps 1 Cup of Spinach ½ Avocado ½ Cup of Steamed Broccoli

WEEK 1

DAY 1

Starting Weight: _____

Breakfast	Fat Flush Drink 3 Boiled Egg Whites ½ Orange or ½ Grapefruit
Lunch	4-5 oz Lean Meat 1-2 Cups Green Vegetables
Snack	Larabar or 10-12 Unsalted Cashews/Almonds with 2 Dates or Prunes or 1 Small Apple and 2 Tsp. Almond Butter
Dinner	4-5 oz Lean Meat 1-2 Cups Green Vegetables

"It's Your Body, Love it." –Unknown

Why did you decide to start this journey?

_____

_____

_____

_____

What goals can you set for yourself to reach by the end of these 30 days?

_____

_____

_____

_____

What did you struggle with today?

_____

_____

_____

_____

What areas can you improve?

_____

_____

_____

_____

DAY 2

Breakfast	Fat Flush Drink
	3 Boiled Egg Whites
	½ Orange or ½ Grapefruit
Lunch	4-5 oz Lean Meat
	1-2 Cups Green Vegetables
Snack	Larabar
	or
	10-12 Unsalted Cashews/Almonds with 2 Dates or Prunes
	or
	1 Small Apple and 2 Tsp. Almond
	Butter
Dinner	4-5 oz Lean Meat
	1-2 Cups Green Vegetables

"You are stronger than the body lets your mind believe. Let your mind tell your body what you can achieve."
–K.M.

How do you plan to resist food temptations?

_____
_____
_____
_____

What did you struggle with today?

_____
_____
_____
_____
_____

What areas can you improve?

_____
_____
_____
_____
_____

DAY 3

Breakfast	Fat Flush Drink
	3 Boiled Egg Whites
	½ Orange or ½ Grapefruit
Lunch	4-5 oz Lean Meat
	1-2 Cups Green Vegetables
Snack	Larabar
	or
	10-12 Unsalted Cashews/Almonds with 2 Dates or Prunes
	or
	1 Small Apple and 2 Tsp. Almond Butter
Dinner	4-5 oz Lean Meat
	1-2 Cups Green Vegetables

"Don't just think you can, know you can and you will."-
K.M.

What are you enjoying about the program so far?

_____

_____

_____

_____

What did you struggle with today?

_____

_____

_____

_____

What areas can you improve?

_____

_____

_____

_____

DAY 4

Breakfast	Fat Flush Drink 3 Boiled Egg Whites 1/2 Cup Oatmeal ¼ Cup of Berries in Oatmeal
Snack	Berry Smoothie
Lunch	4-5 oz Lean Meat 1-2 Cups Green Vegetables
Snack	½ Orange or ½ Grapefruit
Dinner	4-5 oz Lean Meat 1-2 Cups Green Vegetables

"If it doesn't challenge you, it won't change you."
–Fred DeVito

Today is the first day that you can workout on the program if you choose. What are some things you can incorporate to add physical activity into your weekly regimen?

_____

_____

_____

_____

What did you struggle with today?

_____

_____

_____

_____

What areas can you improve?

_____

_____

_____

_____

DAY 5

Breakfast	Fat Flush Drink
	3 Boiled Egg Whites
	½ Orange or ½ Grapefruit
Lunch	3-4 oz Lean Meat
	1-2 Cups Green Vegetables
	½ Cup Grains or ½ Sweet Potato
Snack	Larabar
	or
	10-12 Unsalted Cashews/Almonds with 2 Dates or Prunes
	or
	1 Small Apple and 2 Tsp. Almond
	Butter
Dinner	4-5 oz Lean Meat
	1-2 Cups Green Vegetables

"I've decided that no matter what, this time, I'm not giving up."-K.M.

What good differences can you feel in your body so far?

_____

_____

_____

_____

What did you struggle with today?

_____

_____

_____

_____

What areas can you improve?

_____

_____

_____

_____

DAY 6

Breakfast	Fat Flush Drink
	3 Boiled Egg Whites
	Larabar
	or
	10-12 Unsalted Cashews/Almonds with 2 Dates or Prunes
	or
	1 Small Apple and 2 Tsp. Almond Butter
Snack	Berry Smoothie
Lunch	3-4 oz Lean Meat
	1-2 Cups Green Vegetables
Snack	½ Orange or ½ Grapefruit
Dinner	3-4 oz Lean Meat
	1-2 Cups Green Vegetables

"When you feel like quitting, remember why you started."
-Unknown

What is your WHY? In what way is this healthy journey mandatory instead of optional?

_____

_____

_____

_____

What did you struggle with today?

_____

_____

_____

_____

What areas can you improve?

_____

_____

_____

_____

DAY 7

Breakfast	Berry Smoothie
Snack	1-1.2 oz Dark Chocolate
Lunch	3-4 oz Lean Meat 1-2 Cups Green Vegetables ½ Cup Grains or ½ Sweet Potato
Dinner	3-4 oz Lean Meat 1-2 Cups Green Vegetables 1 Cup Green Tea w/Ginger Root and Lemon Juice *Optional

"Success is the sum of small efforts repeated day in and day out." –Robert Collier

What can you do to guarantee that you succeed in reaching your goals while on this plan?

_____

_____

_____

_____

What did you struggle with today?

_____

_____

_____

_____

What areas can you improve?

_____

_____

_____

_____

END OF WEEK RECAP

What were your non-scale victories?

_____
_____
_____
_____
_____
_____

What health improvements have you seen?

_____
_____
_____
_____
_____

What goals did you make or meet?

_____
_____
_____
_____
_____

WEEK 2

DAY 8

Starting Weight: _____

Breakfast	Fat Flush Drink
	3 Boiled Egg Whites
	½ Orange or ½ Grapefruit
Lunch	4-5 oz Lean Meat
	1-2 Cups Green Vegetables
Snack	Larabar
	or
	10-12 Unsalted Cashews/Almonds with 2 Dates or Prunes
	or
	1 Small Apple and 2 Tsp. Almond
	Butter
Dinner	4-5 oz Lean Meat
	1-2 Cups Green Vegetables

"Motivation is what gets you started, habit is what keeps you going."-Jim Ryun

Are you satisfied with your first weigh in? Why or why not?

_____

_____

_____

_____

What did you struggle with today?

_____

_____

_____

_____

What areas can you improve?

_____

_____

_____

_____

DAY 9

Breakfast	Fat Flush Drink 3 Boiled Egg Whites ½ Orange or ½ Grapefruit
Lunch	3-4 oz Lean Meat 1-2 Cups Green Vegetables ½ Cup Grains or ½ Sweet Potato
Snack	Larabar or 10-12 Unsalted Cashews/Almonds with 2 Dates or Prunes or 1 Small Apple and 2 Tsp. Almond Butter
Dinner	4-5 oz Lean Meat 1-2 Cups Green Vegetables Green Tea

"Today I get to treat myself with everything my body needs. That's my new reward" –M.M.

We don't treat ourselves by rewarding our bodies with foods that are not good for us. What are some healthy treats that you look forward to on the meal plan?

_____

_____

_____

_____

What did you struggle with today?

_____

_____

_____

_____

What areas can you improve?

_____

_____

_____

_____

DAY 10

Breakfast	Fat Flush Drink
	3 Scrambled Egg Whites w/Veggies
	½ Orange or ½ Grapefruit
Lunch	4-5 oz Lean Meat
	1-2 Cups Green Vegetables
Snack	Larabar
	or
	10-12 Unsalted Cashews/Almonds with 2 Dates or Prunes
	or
	1 Small Apple and 2 Tsp. Almond
	Butter
Dinner	4-5 oz Lean Meat
	1-2 Cups Green Vegetables

This month's choices are next month's body." –Unknown

What is your goal for your next weigh in?

_____

_____

_____

_____

What did you struggle with today?

_____

_____

_____

_____

What improvements have you made so far?

_____

_____

_____

_____

DAY 11

Breakfast	Fat Flush Drink
	3 Boiled Egg Whites
	1/2 Cup Oatmeal
	¼ Cup of Berries in Oatmeal
Snack	Berry Smoothie or Apple Smoothie
Lunch	4-5 oz Lean Meat
	1-2 Cups Green Vegetables
Snack	½ Orange or ½ Grapefruit
Dinner	4-5 oz Lean Meat
	1-2 Cups Green Vegetables

"Health is not just for the body but for the mind and soul."-K.M.

Being healthy in your mind is just as important as your body. What are some things that distract you or cause stress during this time of getting healthy? (Eating changes, work, people, finances etc.)

_____

_____

_____

_____

_____

What can you do to minimize distractions and/or stress?

_____

_____

_____

_____

What areas can you improve in your overall health?

_____

_____

_____

_____

DAY 12

Breakfast	Fat Flush Drink 3 Boiled Egg Whites ½ Orange or ½ Grapefruit
Lunch	4-5 oz Lean Meat 1-2 Cups Green Vegetables
Snack	Larabar or 10-12 Unsalted Cashews/Almonds with 2 Dates or Prunes or 1 Small Apple and 2 Tsp. Almond Butter
Dinner	4-5 oz Lean Meat 1-2 Cups Green Vegetables

"Difficult roads often lead to beautiful destinations."
-Unknown

What has been the most difficult thing about getting healthy in the past when it came to starting a new health journey or weight loss journey?

_____

_____

_____

_____

What is different about this plan and this time around that makes you want to keep going?

_____

_____

_____

_____

What areas can you improve?

_____

_____

_____

_____

DAY 13

Breakfast	Fat Flush Drink 3 Boiled Egg Whites Larabar or 10-12 Unsalted Cashews/Almonds with 2 Dates or Prunes or 1 Small Apple and 2 Tsp Almond Butter
Snack	Berry Smoothie or Apple Smoothie
Lunch	3-4 oz Lean Meat 1-2 Cups Green Vegetables
Snack	½ Orange or ½ Grapefruit
Dinner	3-4 oz Lean Meat 1-2 Cups Green Vegetables

"Your health is your real wealth..." -Gandhi

What do you think are the most important benefits of being healthy?

_____

_____

_____

_____

What did you struggle with today?

_____

_____

_____

_____

What areas can you improve?

_____

_____

_____

_____

DAY 14

Breakfast	Berry Smoothie or Apple Smoothie
Snack	1-1.2 oz Dark Chocolate
Lunch	3-4 oz Lean Meat 1-2 Cups Green Vegetables ½ Cup Grains or ½ Sweet Potato
Dinner	3-4 oz Lean Meat 1-2 Cups Green Vegetables 1 Cup Green Tea w/Ginger Root and Lemon Juice *Optional

"Positive thinking and positive eating will lead to positive results." –M.G.

Did you stay on track this week to hit your new weigh in goal? If not, what got you off track?

_____

_____

_____

_____

What did you struggle with today?

_____

_____

_____

_____

What areas can you improve?

_____

_____

_____

_____

END OF WEEK RECAP

What were your non-scale victories?

_____
_____
_____
_____
_____
_____
_____

What health improvements have you seen?

_____
_____
_____
_____
_____
_____

What goals did you make or meet?

_____
_____
_____
_____
_____
_____

WEEK 3

DAY 15

Starting Weight: _____

Breakfast	Fat Flush Drink
	3 Boiled Egg Whites
	½ Orange or ½ Grapefruit
Lunch	4-5 oz Lean Meat
	1-2 Cups Green Vegetables
Snack	Larabar
	or
	10-12 Unsalted Cashews/Almonds with 2 Dates or Prunes
	or
	1 Small Apple and 2 Tsp. Almond
	Butter
Dinner	4-5oz Lean Meat
	1-2 Cups Green Vegetables

"You may not be where you want to be but you are no longer where you used to be. That's progress."-Unknown

What can you do to make this a good week?

_____

_____

_____

_____

What did you struggle with today?

_____

_____

_____

_____

What areas can you improve?

_____

_____

_____

_____

DAY 16

Breakfast	Fat Flush Drink 3 Boiled Egg Whites ½ Orange or ½ Grapefruit
Lunch	3-4 oz Lean Meat 1-2 Cups Green Vegetables ½ Cup Grains or ½ Sweet Potato
Snack	Larabar or 10-12 Unsalted Cashews/Almonds with 2 Dates or Prunes or 1 Small Apple and 2 Tsp. Almond Butter
Dinner	4-5 oz Lean Meat 1-2 Cups Green Vegetables 1 Cup Green Tea w/Ginger Root and Lemon Juice *Optional

"You alone are enough." –Oprah Winfrey

In what way do you compare your life or body to other people?

_____

_____

_____

_____

What did you struggle with today?

_____

_____

_____

_____

What areas can you improve?

_____

_____

_____

_____

DAY 17

Breakfast	Fat Flush Drink 3 Scrambled Egg Whites w/Veggies ½ Orange or ½ Grapefruit
Lunch	4-5 oz Lean Meat 1-2 Cups Green Vegetables
Snack	Larabar or 10-12 Unsalted Cashews/Almonds with 2 Dates or Prunes or 1 Small Apple and 2 Tsp. Almond Butter
Dinner	4-5oz Lean Meat 1-2 Cups Green Vegetables

"Discipline is the bridge between goals and accomplishments." –Jim Rohn

What areas of your health journey do you find it hard to discipline yourself?

_____

_____

_____

_____

What strategies can you use to stay focused and encouraged on the plan?

_____

_____

_____

_____

What unhealthy habits have you broken so far?

_____

_____

_____

_____

DAY 18

Breakfast	Fat Flush Drink
	3 Boiled Egg Whites
	1/2 Cup Oatmeal
	¼ Cup of Berries in Oatmeal
Snack	Berry Smoothie or Apple Smoothie
Lunch	4-5oz Lean Meat
	1-2 Cups Green Vegetables
Snack	½ Orange or ½ Grapefruit
Dinner	4-5 oz Lean Meat
	1-2 Cups Green Vegetables

"Nothing is Impossible, the word itself says, I'm Possible."-Audrey Hepburn

How would your life change if you gave 100 percent effort everyday of this plan?

_____

_____

_____

_____

What did you struggle with today?

_____

_____

_____

_____

What areas can you improve?

_____

_____

_____

_____

DAY 19

Breakfast	Fat Flush Drink 3 Boiled Egg Whites ½ Orange or ½ Grapefruit
Lunch	4-5 oz Lean Meat 1-2 Cups Green Vegetables
Snack	Larabar or 10-12 Unsalted Cashews/Almonds with 2 Dates or Prunes or 1 Small Apple and 2 Tsp. Almond Butter
Dinner	4-5oz Lean Meat 1-2 Cups Green Vegetables

"A goal without a plan is just a wish." -Antoine de Saint-Exupéry

What do you feel is a tangible health goal with this plan?

_____

_____

_____

_____

What did you struggle with today?

_____

_____

_____

_____

What areas can you improve?

_____

_____

_____

_____

DAY 20

Breakfast	Fat Flush Drink
	3 Boiled Egg Whites
	Larabar
	or
	10-12 Unsalted Cashews/Almonds with 2 Dates or Prunes or
	1 Small Apple and 2 Tsp. Almond
	Butter
Snack	Berry Smoothie or Apple Smoothie
Lunch	3-4 oz Lean Meat
	1-2 Cups Green Vegetables
Snack	½ Orange or ½ Grapefruit
Dinner	3-4 oz Lean Meat
	1-2 Cups Green Vegetables

"It's not by coincidence that the word health has heal in it, if you get healthy, you get healing."-M.G.

How else has this plan helped you so far in addition to weight loss?

_____

_____

_____

_____

What did you struggle with today?

_____

_____

_____

_____

What areas can you improve?

_____

_____

_____

_____

DAY 21

Breakfast	Berry Smoothie or Apple Smoothie
Snack	1-1.2 oz Dark Chocolate
Lunch	3-4 oz Lean Meat 1-2 Cups Green Vegetables ½ Cup Grains or ½ Sweet Potato
Dinner	3-4 oz Lean Meat 1-2 Cups Green Vegetables 1 Cup Green Tea w/Ginger Root and Lemon Juice *Optional

"Exercise is a celebration of what your body can do, not a punishment for what you ate." -Unknown

What new activities can you incorporate that makes exercise fun and enjoyable?

_____

_____

_____

_____

What did you struggle with today?

_____

_____

_____

_____

What areas can you improve?

_____

_____

_____

_____

END OF WEEK RECAP

What were your non-scale victories?

_____

_____

_____

_____

_____

_____

What health improvements have you seen?

_____

_____

_____

_____

_____

What goals did you make or meet?

_____

_____

_____

_____

_____

_____

WEEK 4

DAY 22

Starting Weight: _____

Breakfast	Fat Flush Drink
	3 Boiled Egg Whites
	½ Orange or ½ Grapefruit
Lunch	4-5 oz Lean Meat
	1-2 Cups Green Vegetables
Snack	Larabar
	or
	10-12 Unsalted Cashews/Almonds with 2 Dates or Prunes
	or
	1 Small Apple and 2 Tsp. Almond
	Butter
Dinner	4-5oz Lean Meat
	1-2 Cups Green Vegetables

"Excuses don't get results."-Unknown

What excuses, if any, have you made during these last three weeks?

_____

_____

_____

_____

What areas can you improve?

_____

_____

_____

_____

What new recipes can you incorporate to keep your menu interesting?

_____

_____

_____

_____

DAY 23

Breakfast	Fat Flush Drink
	3 Boiled Egg Whites
	½ Orange or ½ Grapefruit
Lunch	3-4 oz Lean Meat
	1-2 Cups Green Vegetables
	½ Cup Grains or ½ Sweet Potato
Snack	Larabar
	or
	10-12 Unsalted Cashews/Almonds with 2 Dates or Prunes
	or
	1 Small Apple and 2 Tsp. Almond
	Butter
Dinner	4-5 oz Lean Meat
	1-2 Cups Green Vegetables
	1 Cup Green Tea w/Ginger Root and Lemon Juice *Optional

"It doesn't get easier, it gets better."- Unknown

How has your life gotten better since starting this plan?

_____

_____

_____

_____

What did you struggle with today?

_____

_____

_____

_____

What areas can you improve?

_____

_____

_____

_____

DAY 24

Breakfast	Fat Flush Drink
	3 Scrambled Egg Whites/Omelette
	w/Veggies
	½ Orange or ½ Grapefruit
Lunch	4-5 oz Lean Meat
	1-2 Cups Green Vegetables
Snack	Larabar
	or
	10-12 Unsalted Cashews/Almonds with 2 Dates or Prunes
	or
	1 Small Apple and 2 Tsp. Almond
	Butter
Dinner	4-5oz Lean Meat
	1-2 Cups Green Vegetables

"Every choice you make has an end result."-Zig Ziglar

What choices have you made while on this plan that have either affected you in a positive way or negative way?

_____

_____

_____

_____

What did you struggle with today?

_____

_____

_____

_____

What areas can you improve?

_____

_____

_____

_____

DAY 25

Breakfast	Fat Flush Drink 3 Boiled Egg Whites 1/2 Cup Oatmeal ¼ Cup of Berries in Oatmeal
Snack	Berry Smoothie or Apple Smoothie
Lunch	4-5oz Lean Meat 1-2 Cups Green Vegetables
Snack	½ Orange or ½ Grapefruit
Dinner	4-5 oz Lean Meat 1-2 Cups Green Vegetables

"Every day is a chance at new beginnings."- M.G.

What have you been most proud of while on this journey to better health?

_____

_____

_____

_____

What did you struggle with today?

_____

_____

_____

_____

What areas can you improve?

_____

_____

_____

_____

DAY 26

Breakfast	Fat Flush Drink
	3 Boiled Egg Whites
	½ Orange or ½ Grapefruit
Lunch	4-5 oz Lean Meat
	1-2 Cups Green Vegetables
Snack	Larabar
	or
	10-12 Unsalted Cashews/Almonds with 2 Dates or Prunes
	or
	1 Small Apple and 2 Tsp. Almond
	Butter
Dinner	4-5 oz Lean Meat
	1-2 Cups Green Vegetables

"All great achievements require time." –Maya Angelou

What is one area that you have been strengthened in since starting this meal plan?

_____

_____

_____

_____

What did you struggle with today?

_____

_____

_____

_____

What areas can you improve?

_____

_____

_____

_____

DAY 27

Breakfast	Fat Flush Drink
	3 Boiled Egg Whites
	Larabar
	or
	10-12 Unsalted Cashews/Almonds with 2 Dates or Prunes
	or
	1 Small Apple and 2 Tsp. Almond Butter
Snack	Berry Smoothie or Apple Smoothie
Lunch	3-4 oz Lean Meat
	1-2 Cups Green Vegetables
Snack	½ Orange or ½ Grapefruit
Dinner	3-4 oz Lean Meat
	1-2 Cups Green Vegetables

"Healthy is not a destination, it's a life journey." –M.G.

What has been the easiest part of this journey?

_____

_____

_____

_____

What is the hardest part of this journey?

_____

_____

_____

_____

Are you on track to reaching your initial goal? If so, what have you done to stay on track. If not, how can you get back on track?

_____

_____

_____

_____

END OF WEEK RECAP

What were your non-scale victories?

_____

_____

_____

_____

_____

_____

What health improvements have you seen?

_____

_____

_____

_____

_____

_____

What permanent lifestyle changes can you implement after the program?

_____

_____

_____

_____

_____

_____

YOU'RE ALMOST THERE!

DAY 28

Breakfast	Berry Smoothie or Apple Smoothie
Snack	1 oz Dark Chocolate
Lunch	3-4 oz Lean Meat 1-2 Cups Green Vegetables ½ Cup Grains or ½ Sweet Potato
Dinner	3-4 oz Lean Meat 1-2 Cups Green Vegetables 1 Cup Green Tea w/Ginger Root and Lemon Juice *Optional

"A strong positive self-image is the best possible preparation for success." -Joyce Brothers

What areas have you gained more confidence in since starting The 30 DD Plan?

_____

_____

_____

_____

What did you struggle with today?

_____

_____

_____

_____

What areas can you improve?

_____

_____

_____

_____

DAY 29

Breakfast	Fat Flush Drink
	3 Boiled Egg Whites
	½ Orange or ½ Grapefruit
Lunch	4-5 oz Lean Meat
	1-2 Cups Green Vegetables
Snack	Larabar
	or
	10-12 Unsalted Cashews/Almonds with 2 Dates or Prunes
	or
	1 Small Apple and 2 Tsp. Almond
	Butter
Dinner	4-5 oz Lean Meat
	1-2 Cups Green Vegetables

"Success isn't about perfection, it's about the right consistency." –M.G.

What parts of the plan have you been the most successful in?

_____

_____

_____

_____

Why did you start this plan?

_____

_____

_____

_____

Why do you think it's important to continue The 30 DD Plan?

_____

_____

_____

_____

What have you learned from previous mistakes made?

_____

_____

_____

_____

IT'S YOUR LAST DAY!

DAY 30

Breakfast	Fat Flush Drink 3 Boiled Egg Whites ½ Orange or ½ Grapefruit
Lunch	3-4 oz Lean Meat 1-2 Cups Green Vegetables ½ Cup Grains or ½ Sweet Potato
Snack	Larabar Or 10-12 Unsalted Cashews/Almonds and 2 Dates or Prunes
Dinner	4-5 oz Lean Meat 1-2 Cups Green Vegetables Green Tea

"Be like a postage stamp. Stick to a thing until you get there." -Josh Billings

How do you plan to stick to a healthy lifestyle after the program is over?

_____

_____

_____

_____

What did you struggle with today?

_____

_____

_____

_____

_____

What areas can you improve?

_____

_____

_____

_____

_____

CONGRATS!

You've completed The 30 Day Difference Clean Eating Plan. Completing this journey is a milestone and the beginning of living healthy, long and strong. This is a huge accomplishment! If you've seen results or benefits, please tell your friends, family and others about this amazing book. We'd love to hear your feedback and how The 30 DD Plan has changed your life. Please submit your testimonial on our website at:

www.30DayDifferenceChallenge.com

For Private Consultations, 1-on-1 Nutrition Coaching or Customized Meal Plans and Recipes please visit:

www.30DayDifferenceChallenge.com/Services

We suggest that you wait at least a full seven days before participating in another round of The 30 DD Plan.

Be on the look out for the Maintenance Phase of The 30 Day Difference Clean Eating Plan. For recipe ideas and healthy inspiration, you can also follow us on Instagram @30DayDifferenceChallenge. Want to share your results on our pages? Be sure to use the hashtag #30DDPlan. Thanks so much for participating. I hope you truly saw a difference. Happy 30 Day!

DAY 31

(Maintenance Day and Final Weigh In)

Ending Weight: _____

Breakfast	Fat Flush Drink
	3 Boiled or Scrambled Egg Whites
	½ Orange or ½ Grapefruit
Lunch	3-4 oz Lean Meat
	1-2 Cups Green Vegetables
	½ Cup Grains or ½ Sweet Potato
Snack	Larabar
	or
	10-12 Unsalted Cashews/Almonds
	and
	2 Dates or Prunes
	or
	1 small apple
	2 Tsp No Sugar Almond Butter
Dinner	4-5 oz Lean Meat
	1-2 Cups Green Vegetables

The 30 Day Difference Clean Eating Plan Results

What was your start weight? _____

What is your end weight? _____

Total Weight Loss: _____

Measurements

How many inches did you lose?

Arms : Start _____   End _____

Chest: Start _____   End_____

Waist: Start _____   End _____

Hips: Start _____   End _____

Thighs: Start _____   End_____

Legs: Start _____   End _____

Dress Size

Shirt Size: Start_____   End_____

Pants Size: Start_____   End _____

References

Carter, Christine. "Please Quit Your Diet, Now." Psychology Today, Sussex Publishers, 2 Mar. 2012, www.psychologytoday.com/blog/raising-happiness/201203/please-quit-your-diet-now.

"Diet." WHO, World Health Organization, Sept. 2014, www.who.int/topics/diet/en/.

Gray, Marlee "Nutrition." F.I.T. Mom Challenge, 1 May 2016, www.fitmomchallenge.co/nutrition.html.

www.brainyquote.com

www.pinterest.com